Quiet Time for the Woman of F

Scripture verses are paraphrased from the King James version of the Holy Bible and World English Bible (WEB) -Public Domain.
Cover and interior design, salutation, coloring pages, scripture selection and arrangement by Cathy Idowu

ISBN 978-0-9801484-7-3 Paperback.

For (Bible study/ women's groups) bulk order, and permissions: Contact:
journalsbycatherine@gmail.com

Cathy Idowu
Ritequest Publishing

Dear *Woman of faith*, thank you for choosing Quiet time for the Woman of Faith as a journal to document your journey and your walk with God. This prayer journal has been designed to help you with your prayer and devotional life, as well as a stress relief tool through the scripture art coloring pages.

Here is something to motivate you as you begin: The Bible gives an account of two sisters named Martha and Mary. Martha kept herself busy with many tasks, but Mary took time out to listen to Jesus' words. In the eyes of Jesus, Mary had chosen the better option, and that choice would not be taken away from her. For us, that would also mean finding time to fellowship with the Lord, through His Word and the Holy Spirit. As compelling as our dawn to dusk to-do lists may be, Jesus gives insight into these daily activities: many are "anxiety-inducing." This is why He said to Martha, "You are anxious about many things, but only one thing is truly needful." So, like Mary, let's treasure the moments we have with Jesus. From this, we'll derive the spirit-sustaining strength and insights to fuel all the other activities that life will send our way.

I hope this journal will end up as a keepsake —full of testimonies of God's faithfulness and treasured memories to pass on to your next generation.

Contents and use of this journal

• Pages highlighting 12 amazing women of the Bible with a section for your notes, if you choose to do an in-depth study on them.

• Pages with scripture affirmation of who you are in Christ accompanied by personally designed beautiful flowers and vases.

• The main journal section is divided into 6 days. Each day includes a "Word for my soul" section —use any devotional, message, or Bible-in-a-year reading, and journal what you sense God is saying to you; An "I'm thankful for" section —include points of gratitude and answered prayer here; A "Prayer focus/ request" section — include any and all types of prayer; A "Letting go of this anxious thought" section— Here's your opportunity to exercise your faith by letting go of anxieties and letting God handle all you bring to Him in prayer.

• At the end of your six days, you have two pages for your seventh day, giving you plenty of space for weekly reflections, ideas, sermon notes, personal or community Bible study or book club notes. In total, you have 12 weeks of journaling pages. Enjoy the journey!

Peace and blessings to you,

Cathy

www.journalsbycatherine.com

This journal belongs to:

_____

Season of Life/ Occasion

_____

Date

_____

"A woman who fears
the Lord is to be
praised."

Proverbs 31:30

Bless the Lord, O my soul, and forgot not all His benefits!

Psalm 103:2

Hannah

"My heart rejoices in the LORD!
The LORD has made me strong. Now
I have an answer for my enemies;
I rejoice because you rescued me.
No one is holy like the LORD!
There is no one besides you;
there is no Rock like our God."

1 Samuel 2 (excerpt)

Deborah

"Hear this, you kings! Listen,
you rulers!
I, even I, will sing to the
LORD;
I will praise the LORD, the
God of Israel, in song
…may all who love you be like
the sun
when it rises in its strength."

Judges 5 (excerpt)

Mary

"My soul magnifies the Lord.
My spirit has rejoiced in God my
Savior,
for he has looked at the humble
state of his servant.
For behold, from now on, all generations will call me blessed.
For he who is mighty has done great
things for me.
Holy is his name.
His mercy is for generations and
generations on those who fear him.
He has shown strength with his arm.
He has scattered the proud in the
imagination of their hearts.
He has put down princes from their
thrones,
and has exalted the lowly.
He has filled the hungry with good
things.
He has sent the rich away empty.
He has given help to Israel, his
servant, that he might remember
mercy,
as he spoke to our fathers,
to Abraham and his offspring for-
ever."

Luke 1:46-55

Love is patient,
love is kind. Love
does not envy, nor is it
proud or rude.
It does not insist on
its own way, nor
does it get easily
offended. It does not
harbor malice.
It does not rejoice in
wrong-doing, but
rejoices in truth.
It bears all things,
believes all things,
hopes all things, and
endures all things.

LOVE NEVER
FAILS.

1 Corinthians 13:4-8

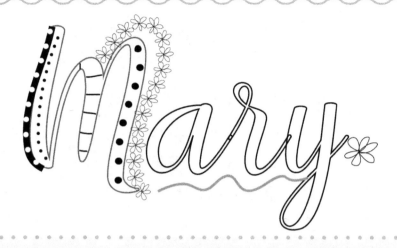

Mary

Mother of Jesus: full of faith, hope, and whole-hearted surrender to the will of God.

Her Story: Luke 1:26-56

Notes

In Christ, you are...

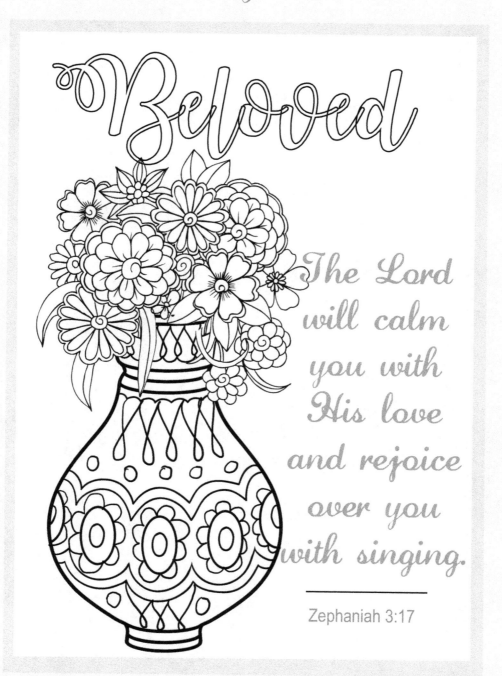

Beloved

The Lord will calm you with His love and rejoice over you with singing.

Zephaniah 3:17

Today's word for my soul

Date:

I'm thankful for...

Letting go of this anxious thought

Prayer focus & requests

Today's word for my soul

Date:

I'm thankful for...

Letting go of this anxious thought

Prayer focus & requests

Today's word for my soul

Date:

I'm thankful for...

Letting go of this anxious thought

Prayer focus & requests

Today's word for my soul

Date:

I'm thankful for...

Letting go of this anxious thought

Prayer focus & requests

Today's word for my soul

Date:

I'm thankful for...

Letting go of this anxious thought

Prayer focus & requests

Today's word for my soul

Date:

I'm thankful for...

Letting go of this anxious thought

Prayer focus & requests

Date: _____

Date: _____

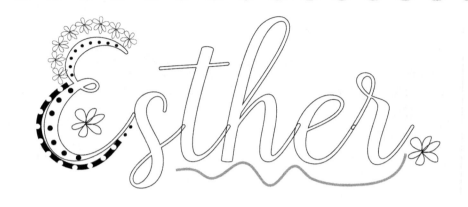

Full of faith and courageous, sensitive to the plight of her people, beautiful with a life-risking purpose.

Her Story: The book of Esther

Notes

In Christ, you are...

Beautiful

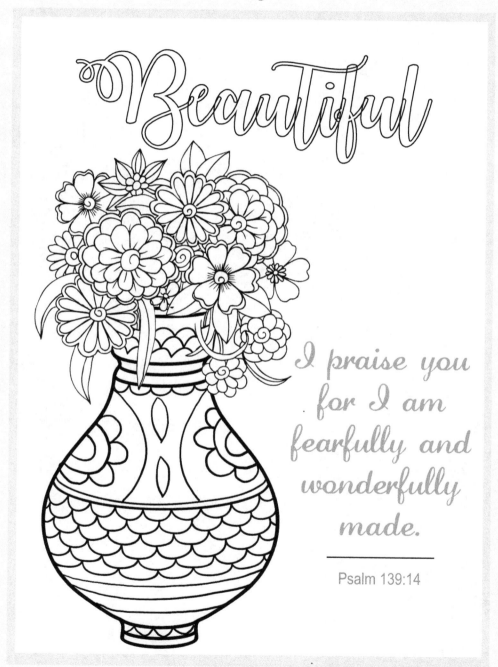

I praise you
for I am
fearfully and
wonderfully
made.

Psalm 139:14

Today's word for my soul

Date:

I'm thankful for...

Letting go of this anxious thought

Prayer focus & requests

Today's word for my soul

Date:

I'm thankful for...

Letting go of this anxious thought

Prayer focus & requests

Today's word for my soul

Date:

I'm thankful for...

Letting go of this anxious thought

Prayer focus & requests

Today's word for my soul

Date:

I'm thankful for...

Letting go of this anxious thought

Prayer focus & requests

Today's word for my soul

Date:

I'm thankful for...

Letting go of this anxious thought

Prayer focus & requests

Today's word for my soul

Date:

I'm thankful for...

Letting go of this anxious thought

Prayer focus & requests

Date: _____

Date: _____

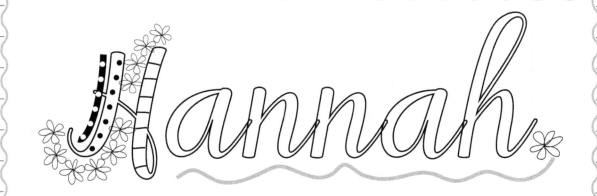

Full of faith and a persevering spirit; focused in mission, and a fervent prayerful, worshipper.

Her Story: 1 Samuel 1-2:11

Notes

In Christ, you are...

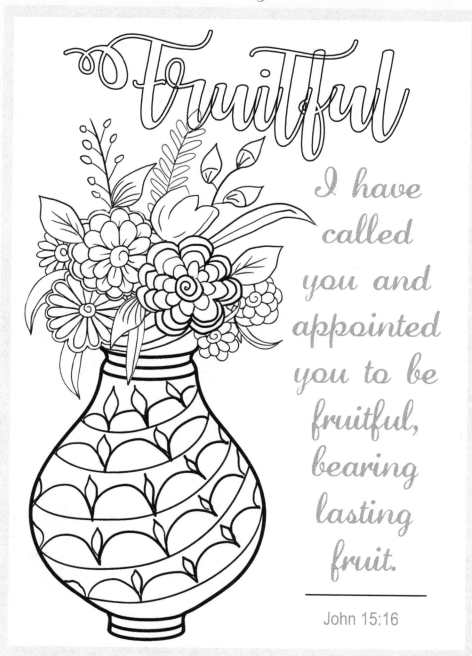

Fruitful

I have called you and appointed you to be fruitful, bearing lasting fruit.

John 15:16

Today's word for my soul

Date:

I'm thankful for...

Letting go of this anxious thought

Prayer focus & requests

Today's word for my soul

Date:

I'm thankful for...

Letting go of this anxious thought

Prayer focus & requests

Today's word for my soul

Date:

I'm thankful for...

Letting go of this anxious thought

Prayer focus & requests

Today's word for my soul

Date:

I'm thankful for...

Letting go of this anxious thought

Prayer focus & requests

Today's word for my soul

Date:

I'm thankful for...

Letting go of this anxious thought

Prayer focus & requests

Today's word for my soul

Date:

I'm thankful for...

Letting go of this anxious thought

Prayer focus & requests

Date: _____

Date: _____

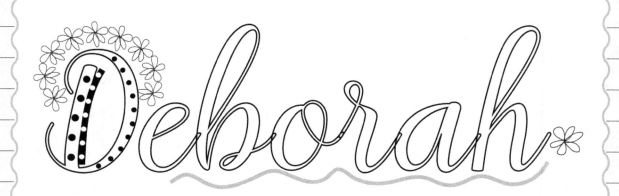

Deborah

Full of faith, wisdom, and foresight; a bold initiator, warrior, and courageous national leader.

Her Story: Judges 4-5

Notes

In Christ, you are...

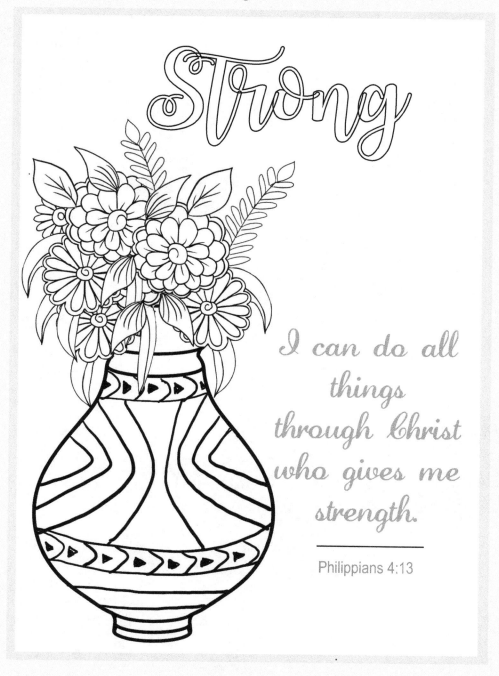

Strong

I can do all
things
through Christ
who gives me
strength.

Philippians 4:13

Today's word for my soul

Date:

I'm thankful for...

Letting go of this anxious thought

Prayer focus & requests

Today's word for my soul

Date:

I'm thankful for...

Letting go of this anxious thought

Prayer focus & requests

Today's word for my soul

Date:

I'm thankful for...

Letting go of this anxious thought

Prayer focus & requests

Today's word for my soul

Date:

I'm thankful for...

Letting go of this anxious thought

Prayer focus & requests

Today's word for my soul

Date:

I'm thankful for...

Letting go of this anxious thought

Prayer focus & requests

Today's word for my soul

Date:

I'm thankful for...

Letting go of this anxious thought

Prayer focus & requests

Date: _____

Date: _____

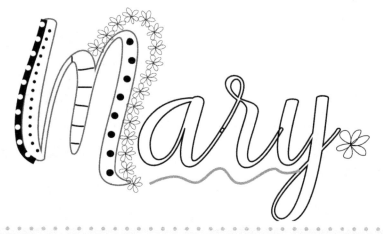

Full of faith and devotion to Jesus, unconcerned about the opinions of others, and extravagant in worship.

Her Story: Luke 7:36-50; John 12:1-8

Notes

In Christ, you are...

Forgiven

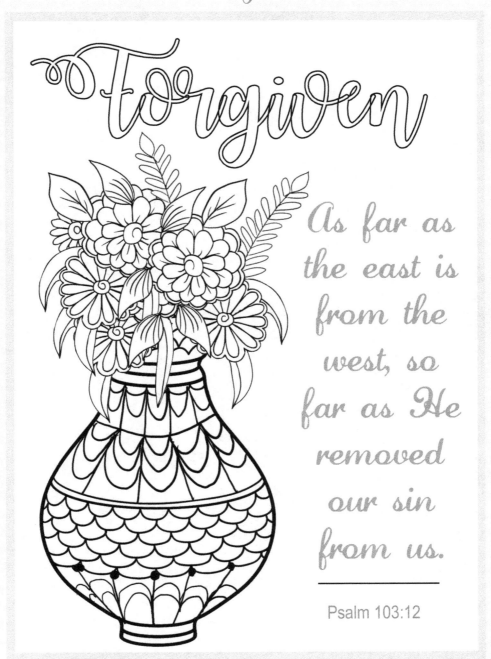

As far as the east is from the west, so far as He removed our sin from us.

Psalm 103:12

Today's word for my soul

Date:

I'm thankful for...

Letting go of this anxious thought

Prayer focus & requests

Today's word for my soul

Date:

I'm thankful for...

Letting go of this anxious thought

Prayer focus & requests

Today's word for my soul

Date:

I'm thankful for...

Letting go of this anxious thought

Prayer focus & requests

Today's word for my soul

Date:

I'm thankful for...

Letting go of this anxious thought

Prayer focus & requests

Today's word for my soul

Date:

I'm thankful for...

Letting go of this anxious thought

Prayer focus & requests

Today's word for my soul

Date:

I'm thankful for...

Letting go of this anxious thought

Prayer focus & requests

Date: _____

Date: _____

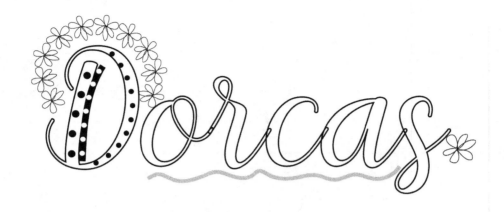

Full of kindness, served with her creative
gifts, and loved by the community of widows.
Her Story: Acts 9:36-42

Notes

In Christ, you are...

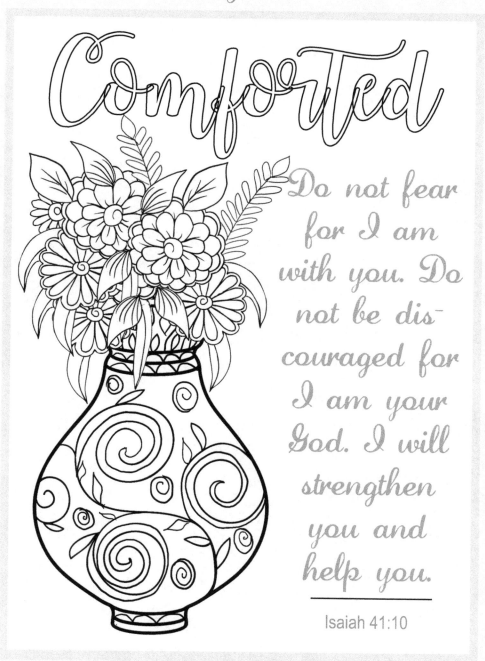

Comforted

Do not fear for I am with you. Do not be discouraged for I am your God. I will strengthen you and help you.

Isaiah 41:10

Today's word for my soul

Date:

I'm thankful for...

Letting go of this anxious thought

Prayer focus & requests

Today's word for my soul

Date:

I'm thankful for...

Letting go of this anxious thought

Prayer focus & requests

Today's word for my soul

Date:

I'm thankful for...

Letting go of this anxious thought

Prayer focus & requests

Today's word for my soul

Date:

I'm thankful for...

Letting go of this anxious thought

Prayer focus & requests

Today's word for my soul

Date:

I'm thankful for...

Letting go of this anxious thought

Prayer focus & requests

Today's word for my soul

Date:

I'm thankful for...

Letting go of this anxious thought

Prayer focus & requests

Date: _____

Date: _____

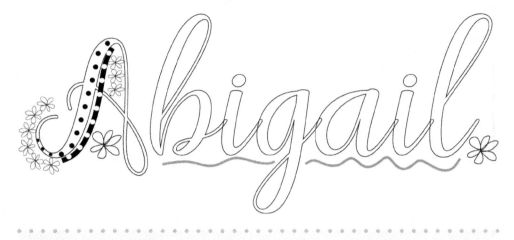

Intelligent in perspective, trusted in her community,
quick to take action, and extravagant in hospitality.

Her Story: 1 Samuel 25:1-42

Notes

In Christ, you are...

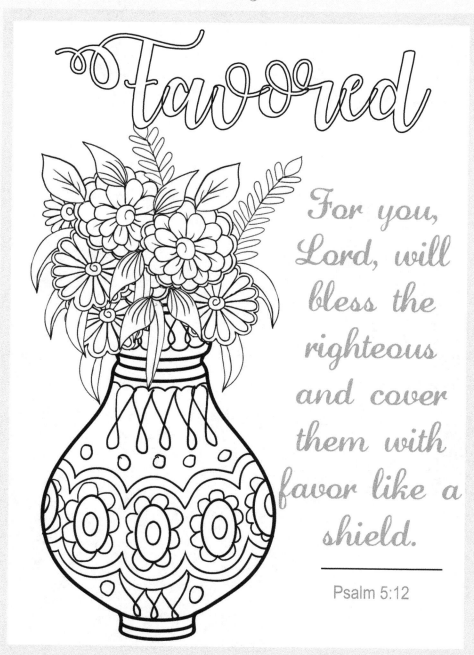

Favored

For you, Lord, will bless the righteous and cover them with favor like a shield.

Psalm 5:12

Today's word for my soul

Date:

I'm thankful for...

Letting go of this anxious thought

Prayer focus & requests

Today's word for my soul

Date:

I'm thankful for...

Letting go of this anxious thought

Prayer focus & requests

Today's word for my soul

Date:

I'm thankful for...

Letting go of this anxious thought

Prayer focus & requests

Today's word for my soul

Date:

I'm thankful for...

Letting go of this anxious thought

Prayer focus & requests

Today's word for my soul

Date:

I'm thankful for...

Letting go of this anxious thought

Prayer focus & requests

Today's word for my soul

Date:

I'm thankful for...

Letting go of this anxious thought

Prayer focus & requests

Date: _____

Date: _____

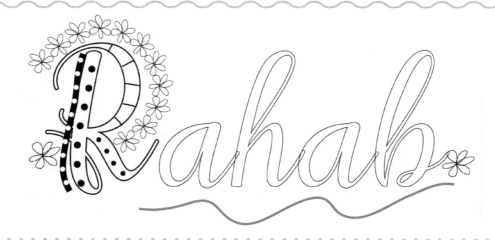

Rahab

Full of faith, courageous in action, stealthy in strategy, and a protector of her household.

Her Story: Joshua 2

Notes

In Christ, you are...

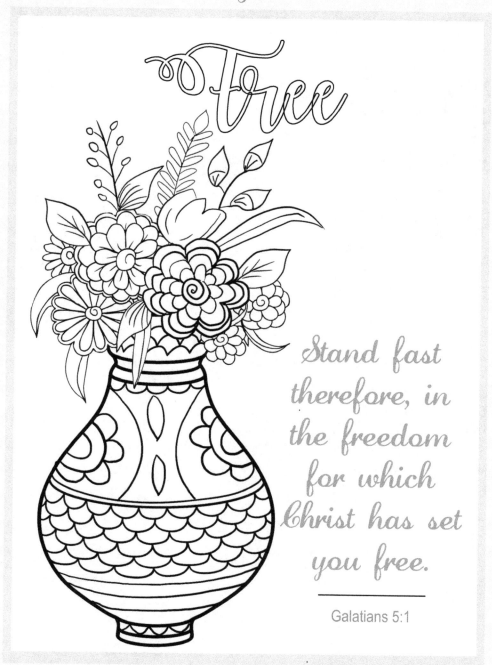

Free

Stand fast therefore, in the freedom for which Christ has set you free.

Galatians 5:1

Today's word for my soul

Date:

I'm thankful for...

Letting go of this anxious thought

Prayer focus & requests

Today's word for my soul

Date:

I'm thankful for...

Letting go of this anxious thought

Prayer focus & requests

Today's word for my soul

Date:

I'm thankful for...

Letting go of this anxious thought

Prayer focus & requests

Today's word for my soul

Date:

I'm thankful for...

Letting go of this anxious thought

Prayer focus & requests

Today's word for my soul

Date:

I'm thankful for...

Letting go of this anxious thought

Prayer focus & requests

Today's word for my soul

Date:

I'm thankful for...

Letting go of this anxious thought

Prayer focus & requests

Date: _____

Date: _____

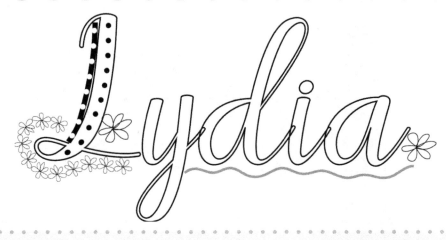

Full of faith, successful in business, persuasive, and extravagant in showing hospitality

Her Story: Acts 16:13-15

Notes

In Christ, you are...

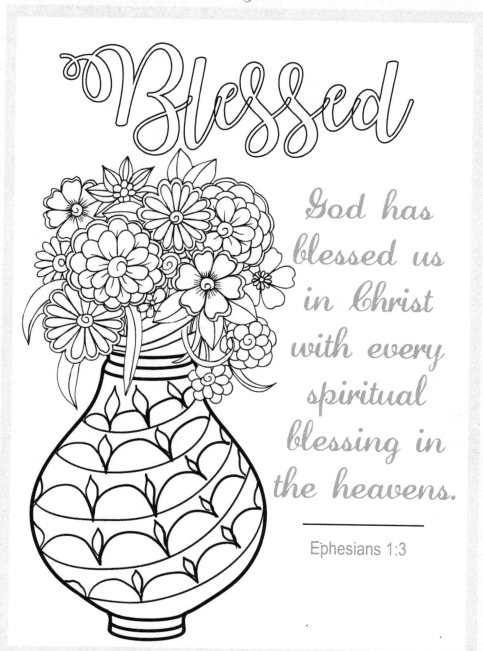

Blessed

God has
blessed us
in Christ
with every
spiritual
blessing in
the heavens.

Ephesians 1:3

Today's word for my soul

Date:

I'm thankful for...

Letting go of this anxious thought

Prayer focus & requests

Today's word for my soul

Date:

I'm thankful for...

Letting go of this anxious thought

Prayer focus & requests

Today's word for my soul

Date:

I'm thankful for...

Letting go of this anxious thought

Prayer focus & requests

Today's word for my soul

Date:

I'm thankful for...

Letting go of this anxious thought

Prayer focus & requests

Today's word for my soul

Date:

I'm thankful for...

Letting go of this anxious thought

Prayer focus & requests

Today's word for my soul

Date:

I'm thankful for...

Letting go of this anxious thought

Prayer focus & requests

Date: _____

Date: _____

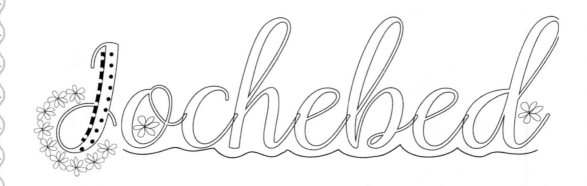

The mother of Moses: Strong in faith and hope,
a risk-taker, and courageous in oppression.
Her Story: Numbers 26:59, Exodus 2:1-8

Notes

In Christ, you are...

Bold

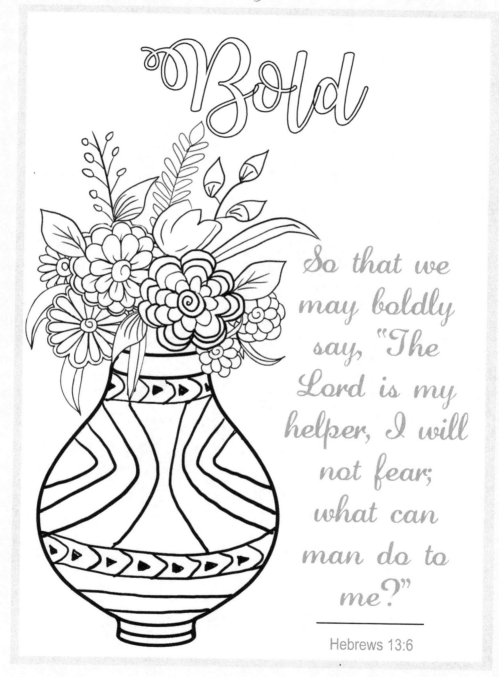

So that we may boldly say, "The Lord is my helper, I will not fear; what can man do to me?"

Hebrews 13:6

Today's word for my soul

Date:

I'm thankful for...

Letting go of this anxious thought

Prayer focus & requests

Today's word for my soul

Date:

I'm thankful for...

Letting go of this anxious thought

Prayer focus & requests

Today's word for my soul

Date:

I'm thankful for...

Letting go of this anxious thought

Prayer focus & requests

Today's word for my soul

Date:

I'm thankful for...

Letting go of this anxious thought

Prayer focus & requests

Today's word for my soul

Date:

I'm thankful for...

Letting go of this anxious thought

Prayer focus & requests

Today's word for my soul

Date:

I'm thankful for...

Letting go of this anxious thought

Prayer focus & requests

Date: _____

Date: _____

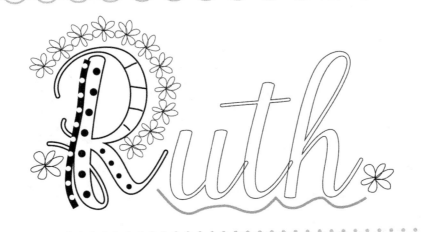

Committed in love, full of hope, and dedicated in her pursuit of a holy legacy.

Her Story: The book of Ruth

Notes

In Christ, you are...

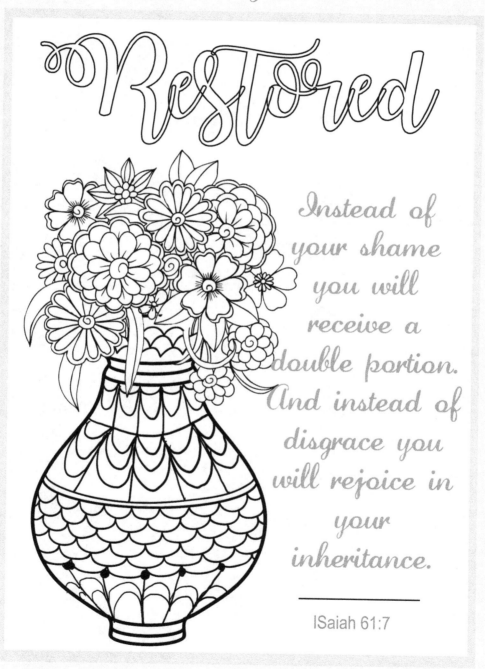

Restored

Instead of your shame you will receive a double portion. And instead of disgrace you will rejoice in your inheritance.

ISaiah 61:7

Today's word for my soul

Date:

I'm thankful for...

Letting go of this anxious thought

Prayer focus & requests

Today's word for my soul

Date:

I'm thankful for...

Letting go of this anxious thought

Prayer focus & requests

Today's word for my soul

Date:

I'm thankful for...

Letting go of this anxious thought

Prayer focus & requests

Today's word for my soul

Date:

I'm thankful for...

Letting go of this anxious thought

Prayer focus & requests

Today's word for my soul

Date:

I'm thankful for...

Letting go of this anxious thought

Prayer focus & requests

Today's word for my soul

Date:

I'm thankful for...

Letting go of this anxious thought

Prayer focus & requests

Date: _____

Date: _____

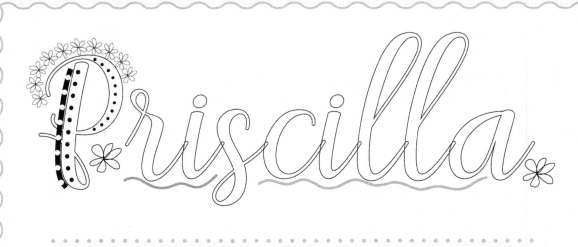

Full of faith and in the knowledge of God's word; committed to the spread and teaching of the gospel.

Her Story: Acts 18:18-26

Notes

In Christ, you are...

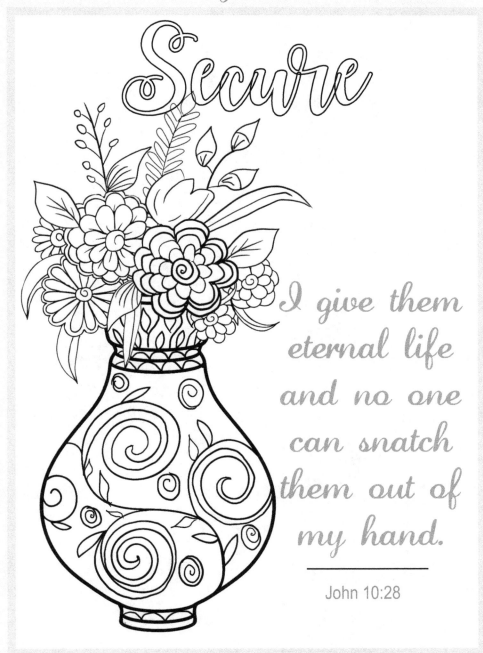

Secure

I give them
eternal life
and no one
can snatch
them out of
my hand.

John 10:28

Today's word for my soul

Date:

I'm thankful for...

Letting go of this anxious thought

Prayer focus & requests

Today's word for my soul

Date:

I'm thankful for...

Letting go of this anxious thought

Prayer focus & requests

Today's word for my soul

Date:

I'm thankful for...

Letting go of this anxious thought

Prayer focus & requests

Today's word for my soul

Date:

I'm thankful for...

Letting go of this anxious thought

Prayer focus & requests

Today's word for my soul

Date:

I'm thankful for...

Letting go of this anxious thought

Prayer focus & requests

Today's word for my soul

Date:

I'm thankful for...

Letting go of this anxious thought

Prayer focus & requests

Date: _____

Date: _____

Other journals by Journals by Catherine

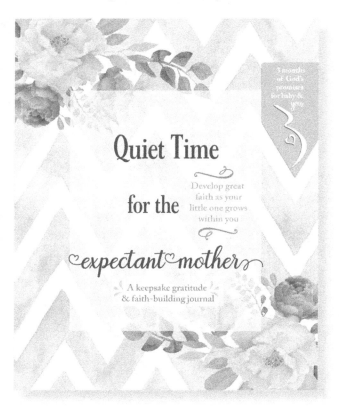

Quiet Time for the Expectant Mother

ISBN 978-0980148466

This is the perfect gift for a first time mom-to-be who is a woman of faith. So, gift this to yourself, a friend, co-worker, sister or daughter. It works well as a pregnancy planner, diary and prayer journal all in one, whether you're a mom-to-be of one or even expecting multiples. This season is full of your most amazing expectation - sometimes joyful, but admit it, sometimes filled with anxiety. This prayer journal has been designed to meet your heartfelt needs, in all of these circumstances.

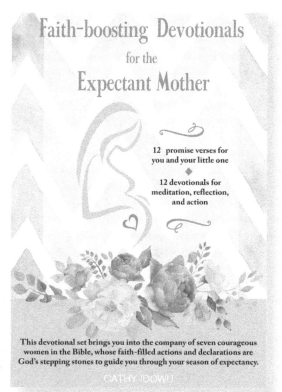

Faith-boosting Devotionals for the Expectant Mother

A Kindle book based on devotions in the Quiet Time for the Expectant Mother journal.

ASIN B07P71G821

Faith-building Devotions for the Expectant Mother is based on the faith and courage of seven women in the Bible. It is specifically tailored towards the needs of a faith-focused expectant mother, who is seeking encouragement in her walk of faith while pregnant.

...et Time for the Bride to Be

ISBN 978-0980148428

...his is an excellent gift response to ...our friend's, sister's or daughter's engagement or, maybe even yours! Planning a wedding can be quite stressful, so be deliberate about creating quiet time. Quiet Time for the Bride to Be meets the need of the Christian bride-to-be seeking to journal memories during this special season.

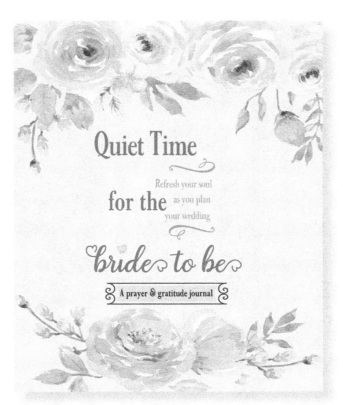

Quiet Time
for the
Refresh your soul
as you plan
your wedding
bride to be
A prayer & gratitude journal

Thank you!

I'm delighted you chose my journal. Whether you've received it as a gift or purchased it for yourself, I hope you're enjoying your experience with it. I'd also appreciate it if you could take a moment to spread your happy experience with others, by leaving a review on Amazon or your online bookstore. Thank you!!

Much blessings,
Cathy

CPSIA information can be obtained
at www.ICGtesting.com
Printed in the USA
LVHW012251071019
633403LV00003B/1388/P